Anti-Inflammatory Diet Guide

The Guide To Reduce Inflammation And Live A Healthy Life Without Pain

LELA GIBSON

LELA GIBSON

CONTENTS

Introduction

I want to thank you and congratulate you for buying the book, *"Anti-Inflammatory Diet Guide"*.

This book contains proven steps and strategies on how to reduce inflammation and live a healthy life without pain.

Each day, we expose our bodies to chemicals, processed foods high in additives and other unhealthy ingredients as well as other pollutants. It is no wonder that suffering from inflammation is quite common.

For most people, the first thing they do once they discover that they are suffering from inflammation is to reach for drugs. However, the thing about drugs is that they address the symptoms associated with inflammation. Therefore, if you want to deal with the problem, you need to address the root cause of inflammation. One of the main causes of inflammation is our diet.

In this book, you will learn more about inflammation and the anti-inflammatory diet that you need to embrace if you want to treat inflammation.

Be sure to like us on Facebook.

Thanks again for buying this book, I hope you enjoy it!

Inflammation: A Comprehensive Overview

Inflammation: What Is It?

Inflammation is the biological response your body goes into when dealing with harmful stimuli such as irritants, pathogens, or even damaged cells. In simple terms, it is a self-protection mechanism that allows your body to begin the healing process.

The term inflammation actually comes from the Latin word 'inflamino' that means 'set alight' or 'ignited'. The 'hotness' or 'inflammation' you feel after you cut yourself or injure yourself is the result of your body working hard to heal itself. However, at some point, inflammation can result in even more inflammation as a response to the already existing inflammation; this can become self-perpetuating hence worsening the problem.

What happens when your body experiences 'too much' inflammation? To understand that, we need to look at the various types of inflammation:

Types of Inflammation

When referring to inflammation, there are two main types outlined below:

1. *Acute inflammation*

This type of inflammation starts rapidly and usually occurs over a short period (within a couple of minutes, lasting up to a few days). This kind of inflammation may occur in instances such as when you suffer from a sore throat from singing, cut, or scrape your skin, tonsillitis, or even an instance where you sprain your ankle. In such a case, you will experience pain, swelling, and redness as a response by your body to repair itself. Acute inflammation usually reduces as soon as the tissue heals.

The main symptoms of acute inflammation are quite obvious. They include;

Pain: The inflamed area will be painful especially to the touch. The pain is a result of the release of chemicals that stimulate nerve endings. This in turn makes the area more sensitive.

Redness: This usually happens because capillaries in that area fill with blood more than usual.

Immobility: You may experience numbness or loss of function in the injured area

Swelling: This happens because of fluid accumulation in the injured area

Heat: Because of blood present in the affected area, you will experience hotness on touching.

2. *Chronic inflammation*

On the other hand, chronic inflammation (also referred to as systemic inflammation) may last a couple of months or even longer. In this case, the symptoms are not so obvious. Since this kind of inflammation lasts longer, it may result in progressive and severe tissue damage and lead to inflammatory diseases. Chronic inflammation develops in response to autoimmune diseases, environmental and habitual factors, and conditions such as osteoarthritis

Some of the telltale signs of chronic inflammation include; rashes, joint pain, fatigue, gum disease, weight gain, brain fog and frequent headaches, mood issues, bloating & other digestive problems.

Inflammation Causes and Risk Factors

Many factors can increase your risks of suffering from chronic inflammation). Below are some of these factors;

1. Excessive weight

When you have excessive weight, an inflammatory response occurs in from within fat cells. This is especially true with age. As fat tissues age, they promote inflammation. This therefore means that younger, obese people are less likely to suffer from inflammation than their older counterparts are.

2. Stress

Like inflammation, stress can be chronic or acute. Acute stress is normal while chronic stress is unhealthy. Acute stress helps you respond to external factors such when a dog chases you. This stress will help you run faster. On the other hand, chronic stress is long term and can develop from bad experiences such as work anxiety or a failing marriage.

When you undergo stress, the body releases cortisol hormone into your bloodstream; cortisol is also responsible for keeping inflammatory response in check. However, chronic stress can dampen the hormone's ability to keep inflammatory response in check hence increasing the possibility of a chronic inflammation.

Chronic stress can also increase production of inflammatory white blood cells hence increasing risk of diseases related to inflammation.

3. Smoking

The smoke from cigarettes irritates the lungs. This can lead to a small level of inflammation that can then worsen already existing lung-related problems such as allergies and COPD. The inflammation and chronic injuries to the lungs caused by smoking can also result in cell mutation, which can lead to lung cancer.

Smoking also increases some contributors of inflammation such as the increase of white blood cells and C-reactive protein (produced by the liver). Nicotine also activates neutrophil, a kind of white blood cell that causes tissue damage because of excessive inflammation. In turn, this leads to even more inflammation as a response hence creating a cycle. Note that in normal situations, Neutrophils work to protect the body.

4. Gut bacteria

Did you know that 70% of your body's immune cells are in your intestines? This means that gut bacteria can affect your immunity. These bacteria can either activate inflammation or suppress it depending on what they are. This is why there is a lot of interest on how probiotics influence the response of inflammation in the gut. The inflammatory diet in this case works to reduce gut inflammation hence reducing the risk of chronic inflammation.

5. Consumption of alcohol

When you drink alcohol, the liver breaks down the alcohol. After completing the process, there is release of toxic by-products. These products promote inflammation. Heavy drinking can lead to a fatty liver (steatosis), a condition where fat accumulates in liver. At this point, you might suffer from liver inflammation thus resulting in cirrhosis or hepatitis.

6. The use of oral contraceptives

According to research conducted by PLOS ONE in 2014, women who take oral contraceptives have a higher risk of suffering from low grade inflammation than women who do not. This is attributed to the increase in the release of C-reactive protein which is an inflammation marker.

So what happens if you suffer from inflammation? What's the worst that can happen?

Effects of inflammation

A little inflammation (acute inflammation) is not a bad thing. In fact, when it happens, you should rejoice in knowing that your body is working tirelessly to correct the situation. However, like most good things, inflammation can get out of hand (chronic inflammation). When this happens, you may experience various health complications such as:

Weight Gain

Every day, thousands of people try to lose weight to no avail. They complain that they've tried out various diets but somehow none seem to be working. If they do find something that works, sooner than later, they are back to gaining the weight they thought they'd lost. This is because they neglect to look into inflammation as the cause for their weight gain. Inflammation contributes to weight gain in various ways. These include:

- If inflammation happens in the brain, it interferes with the functioning of the hypothalamus and this in turn increases your appetite and slows down your metabolism. When this happens, you will be eating a lot but burning up less energy, which leads to weight gain.

- Gut inflammation leads to leptin and insulin resistance. Leptin is the satiety hormone that tells your brain when you have had enough. When suffering from leptin resistance, you just eat and eat some more before leptin can communicate that you have had enough, which leads to weight gain. Another thing that gut inflammation does is to increase intestinal permeability. When this happens, more toxins will be able to permeate your bloodstream. Usually toxins are stored in fat cells to remove them from circulation. The more toxins you have, the more the fat cells expand to accommodate the more toxins leading to weight gain.

- Inflammation in the endocrine system suppresses adrenal and thyroid function. One of the main functions of the adrenal gland is to burn fat. Therefore, when you suppress the functioning of the adrenal gland, you are unable to burn fat, as you should leading to weight gain.

As you have read, inflammation is bad for you if you want to maintain the ideal weight.

Metabolic Syndrome

Metabolic syndrome refers to a group/cluster of lifestyle-related diseases including cardiovascular disease and obesity. They are clustered together because all of these diseases are linked to metabolic dysfunction. Markers of metabolic dysfunction include:

- Central obesity – this is excessive tummy fat

- Hyperinsulinaemia – this refers to ongoing high levels of insulin

- Insulin resistance –your body loses sensitivity to insulin (you need more insulin to manage your blood sugar levels)

But the question is how these three factors are connected. Well, when on a diet high in carbohydrates, your blood sugar levels increase leading to high insulin levels to help blood cells absorb the glucose and thus manage your blood sugar levels. When you have high insulin levels, the production of cytokines (which are pro-inflammatory) increases and in turn this causes inflammation especially in predisposed persons. Once inflammation increases, it brings with it an increase in the production of free radicals. Free radicals affect cellular functions and one of those functions just happens to be insulin sensitivity. This is why chronic low-grade inflammation is linked to all three markers; that is, raised insulin levels, obesity and decreased insulin sensitivity.

Chronic Fatigue

Many people suffering from chronic fatigue have been told that the disease 'is all in their minds'. Fortunately, in recent years more researchers have began looking into the association of chronic fatigue and inflammation. This is mainly because the two possess many similar symptoms including muscular pain and tenderness, sore throat, joint pain, swollen lymph nodes and sore throat.

As you know, inflammation is the way your body reacts to foreign particles. When you have symptoms of inflammation, it is safe to say that your body is fighting something even if that something is not yet known. This is why researchers link an overactive immune system to chronic fatigue.

Another thing that associates chronic fatigue with inflammation is the lack of cortisol in patients suffering from chronic fatigue. Cortisol is known to suppress inflammation. Thus, if your body has a cortisol deficiency, it will not be able to suppress inflammation and this will worsen symptoms of chronic fatigue. A dietary change often helps people suffering from chronic fatigue.

Heart disease

Chronic inflammation and cardiovascular diseases have a very close connection. This is because of the depositing of cholesterol in blood vessels, which in turn acts as a catalyst. Blood, on the other hand, has cytokines that deal with these insults hence leading to systemic inflammation. Growing fatty plaque and inflamed blood vessels can result in blood clots and blockages that can then lead to heart attacks.

People who suffer from chronic inflammation because of an autoimmune disorder are at a higher risk of suffering from heart attacks. In addition, researchers have discovered that bacteria from gum disease can absorb into the blood vessels and heart. The bacteria can act as a catalyst hence leading to inflammation. This in turn increases your risk of suffering from a heart attack.

Some types of arthritis

When you hear the name arthritis, you automatically associate it with pain. Well, it is no coincidence since arthritis refers to inflammation in joints. When your joints experience inflammation, you will feel pain. The types of arthritis that have been linked to inflammation include:

- Gouty arthritis

- Rheumatoid arthritis

- Psoriatic arthritis

- Systematic lupus erythematosus

When you suffer from these types of arthritis, you may experience inflammation symptoms such as redness, joint stiffness, swelling of the joints, pain in the joints and loss of joint function.

It is important to note that inflammation does not have to be painful for it to be present. This is because many organs in your body just don't have enough pain-sensitive areas for you to feel that inflammatory sensation. This means that you can suffer from chronic inflammation over time without knowing, only for you to experience the effects of inflammation.

It is also important to note that various things can cause inflammation including:

- Processed foods high in sugar and unhealthy fats

- Omega-6 fats (and not enough Omega-3 fatty acids)

- Sleep deprivation

- Chronic stress

- Smoking

- Pollution

- Environmental chemicals

- Lack of exercise

Thus, chances are, if you experience any of the above things, you may be suffering from inflammation whether or not you experience pain.

The first thing you should do once you notice that you suffer from inflammation is not to reach for drugs because drugs just address the symptoms and not the root cause but rather to make some lifestyle changes. This is because most of the causes of inflammation can be addressed by making lifestyle changes like exercising more, reducing exposure to pollutants, not smoking and dietary changes.

In this book, we will focus on addressing inflammation by adopting an anti-inflammatory diet. Let us learn more about anti-inflammatory diet in the next chapter.

Anti-Inflammatory Diet: The Solution To Inflammation

An anti-inflammatory diet is a diet that is designed to reduce inflammation. Unlike most diets, it is not a one-size-fits-all diet. But it does include the dos and don'ts to guide you on how to proceed.

This means, it is up to you to check out the 'dos' or foods that have anti-inflammatory properties so that you can customize the diet according to your needs. For example, the diet recommends eating whole grains including wheat. However, some people don't react well to gluten. This means, they may not include gluten in their diet. However, they can certainly include other foods on the allowed foods list.

Other foods that have anti-inflammatory properties include fruits, vegetables, beans and foods that contain Omega-3s. You should also avoid foods that have inflammatory properties like highly processed foods, foods high in sugar and unhealthy fats.

It is important to point out that the anti-inflammatory diet is not a diet per say but rather a lifestyle change. You will be making a conscious decision to reduce the sources of inflammation. Let us learn more about how an anti-inflammatory diet will help address inflammation.

How An Anti-Inflammatory Diet Suppresses Inflammation

It is important to understand how the anti-inflammatory diet works in order to be motivated to adopt the diet. Several related things affect inflammation. These are:

Free radicals

As you know, the human body is composed of cells. In turn, these cells are composed of molecules. The molecules consist of atoms. These atoms have elements joined by chemical bonds. The strength of the bonds determines the stability of the molecules.

Weak bonds often split leading to 'free radicals' that can quickly react with other compounds in order to gain stability. In the course of doing this, the free radicals can displace other molecules, 'stealing' their electrons and this can lead to a chain reaction that can cause disastrous effects by disrupting a living cell.

It is important to note that while free radicals are formed normally during metabolism, certain factors such as eating certain foods, daily stress, processed foods, smoking, pollution, drugs, some herbicides and radiation can also lead to the spawning of free radicals. When the free radicals become too many, it leads to oxidative stress.

Oxidative stress

Your body is built in such a way that it neutralizes and processes free radicals. Unfortunately, when the free radicals are too many, your body will be unable to neutralize them. It will become overwhelmed and this will create an imbalance. This imbalance is what it referred to as oxidative stress and it leads to inflammation.

Inflammation

Many experts suspect that oxidative stress is responsible for starting a bio-chemical cascade that leads to inflammation and other degenerative diseases. Remember I mentioned earlier that free radicals could overwhelm the system.

Think of your body like a computer. You can use it to perform many tasks. When you open one or two programs or documents, you have no trouble performing the tasks that will lead to getting the outcome you desire. However, what happens when you open 10 or more programs to deal with various tasks? Suddenly your computer becomes too slow. It becomes overheated.

The same can happen to your body if it has too many radicals. It becomes inflamed. When this happens, you will need antioxidants to bring down the inflammation. This is where the anti-inflammatory diet comes in.

Antioxidants

Antioxidants, which can be found in various antioxidant rich foods, work well to trap or neutralize free radicals. Antioxidants 'donate' their electrons such that free radicals are forced to bond to them. This stops the electron stealing reaction. It also protects cells from the damage caused by free radicals 'stealing' their electrons.

When free radicals are too many, they wreak havoc in your body. They cause damage and lead to oxidative stress, which leads to inflammation. Thus, neutralizing free radicals is the key to reducing inflammation. An anti-inflammatory diet contains many foods that are rich in antioxidants that can effectively reduce inflammation.

In summary, an anti-inflammatory diet does away with foods that cause oxidative stress while encouraging you to eat foods rich in antioxidants. When you follow this diet, you will effectively neutralize free radicals, prevent oxidative stress and consequently reduce inflammation. This is why it is important to know what to eat and what not to eat.

Anti-Inflammatory Diet: What To Eat

As we've seen, various things can trigger inflammation. There is no reason you should add on to this by eating foods that cause inflammation. In fact, by eating anti-inflammatory foods you can help your body deal with inflammation. Below are some anti-inflammatory foods that you should include in your diet

Fruits and Vegetables

Fruits and vegetables are rich in anti-inflammatory antioxidants and should feature prominently in your diet. Below are some of the best fruits and vegetables for treating inflammation:

Dark, leafy greens

Dark, leafy greens such as kale, romaine and spinach are great for reducing inflammation because they are rich in antioxidants. Kale contains quercetin and Kaempferol antioxidants while romaine contains carotenoids and spinach contains the antioxidant lutein. They are also equipped with other anti-inflammatory agents. You can enjoy such vegetables in salads and smoothies.

Blueberries

Fruits have anti-inflammatory vitamins, Vitamin A, Vitamin C and Vitamin E. These are great at helping your body repair itself. Blueberries also contain the powerful antioxidant anthocyanin, which is great for fighting inflammation. Eat the berries as a snack or add them to your salad and smoothies.

Cruciferous veggies

Cruciferous veggies such as broccoli, cabbage, kale and cauliflower are loaded with antioxidants such as lutein, zeaxanthin and carotenoids. This means they can successfully reduce inflammation and the symptoms associated with it. Make it a habit to increase your consumption of such vegetables. You can even include them in juices and smoothies.

Avocados

Avocados are great for reducing inflammation because they are high in carotenoids. Carotenoids fight inflammation. However, as always, you need to be careful when consuming avocados. Don't overdo it. Half a medium avocado per day should be enough for you. Anymore and you'll start adding on the pounds. You can eat it, as it is, add it to your salad or make guacamole if you'd like.

Asparagus

Asparagus is said to be a super anti-inflammatory food. This is because it has various anti-inflammatory nutrients such as asparanin A, quercetin, diosgenin, rutin, protodioscin, isorhamnetin, kaempferol and sarsasapogenin. Asparagus also has antioxidants. This makes it very useful in the fight against inflammation.

Beetroot

Beetroot is another important food you should include in your diet. It has anti-inflammatory benefits along other properties. Beetroot has phytonutrients such as isobetanin, betanin and vulgaxanthin that are linked to heart health. As you know by now, heart disease is also categorized as a symptom of chronic inflammation. You can include beetroot in salads and juices.

Herbs and Spices

Ginger

Ginger is a well-known spice among chefs. Apart from adding flavour to foods and tea, it is used for its healing properties. It contains anti-oxidants which are also good at fighting inflammation. You can sprinkle a dash of ginger onto your tea and soups whenever you like. This will increase your consumption of this useful spice.

Garlic

Garlic has been linked to various health benefits such as cardiovascular health and prevention of obesity and arthritis. It also has anti-inflammatory properties. Garlic contains the compounds thiacremonone and vinyldithin, which are good at inhibiting inflammatory messenger molecules. Allicin, a compound in garlic, also has many anti-inflammatory benefits. You can use garlic in various foods, salads and soups.

Turmeric

Turmeric is a chef's best friend because it not only adds flavour to food but it also adds colour. Another thing it is known for is its anti-inflammatory properties. You can put it in your vegetables and soup. But take note that turmeric is a bit pungent. If you're not used to it, start with using a little at a time and gradually increase the content.

Whole Grains

Fiber is known to help fight inflammation. Whole grains are high in fiber. Eat foods high in fiber such as brown rice, oatmeal and whole-wheat bread. However, you should be careful to ensure that your body does not react negatively to the gluten contained in wheat.

Beans and Nuts

Beans are also high in fiber and they have antioxidants. They also contain other anti-inflammatory properties that will prove quite useful to you. Nuts are also good for reducing inflammation. They are high in healthy fats that work to stop inflammation. A handful of nuts per day should be enough for you.

Foods Rich in Omega 3

Omega 3 fatty acids are great in fighting inflammation. Flaxseed contains this fatty acid and is especially good for the cardiovascular system. It also serves as a building block for molecules that work to prevent inflammation. Apart from that, omega 3 has been shown to prevent inflammation-based diseases such as depression, inflammatory bowel syndrome, diabetes, heart disease, asthma, osteoporosis and rheumatoid arthritis.

Apart from eating flaxseed, you should also eat fish and seafood. Endeavour to eat at least two servings each week. Herring sardines and salmon should feature in your diet as well as walnuts.

Chia seeds are also high in omega-3 fatty acids. You can add chia seeds to your salads and soups.

Supplements

You can also take supplements to reduce inflammation. These include:

- Spirulina – these algae is known for its strong antioxidant effects. It works to reduce inflammation and strengthen the immune system. You just need to take 1-8 grams per day.

- Resveratrol – this antioxidant can be found in fruits with purple skin such as blueberries and grapes. It is used to reduce inflammation in people who suffer from gastritis, heart disease, ulcerative colitis and insulin resistance. Take 150-500mg in a day.

- Ginger – ginger can also be taken in supplement form. You only need to take 1-2 grams in a day.

- Curcumin – this is found in turmeric and is great at reducing inflammation. You can take up to 100-500mg of this supplement per day.

- Fish oil – you can take fish oil especially if you don't eat fish regularly. Fish oil contains the beneficial omega-3 fatty acids which decrease inflammation. Take 1-1.5 grams of fish oil supplements per day.

Before taking any supplements, you need to read the instructions carefully to ensure the supplements do not interfere with any medicines you are already taking.

Good Fat

You should be careful about the fats you consume. Stick to coconut oil, hemp seeds, avocados, extra-virgin oil, organic canola oil and oily cold water fish such as trout, tuna, salmon and mackerel.

Fiber Rich Food

Foods high in fiber are also great at reducing inflammation. You can eat foods such as barley, quinoa, okra, brown rice, lima beans, black beans, almonds, eggplant, lentils, acorn squash, figs, chia seeds and berries.

Vitamin D

Another thing you should not neglect is vitamin D. This important vitamin often comes up when people are talking about things such as bone health and winter blues. Lack of vitamin D can quickly put you in a gloomy mood. This vitamin is also important when it comes to treating inflammation. Most people suffering from inflammatory conditions are often diagnosed with low vitamin D; therefore the importance of eating foods rich in vitamin D.

Apart from consuming anti-inflammatory foods rich in vitamin D, you can also get your daily dose from the natural sun. This means basking in the sun during morning and evening hours. The best time to do this is between eight and ten in the morning and four and six in the afternoon. This will allow you to enjoy the sun without fear of your skin being damaged by harmful sun rays.

If you live in an area that doesn't have much sun, you need to get creative. For example, if you live in an apartment complex, you will need to go outside and walk in the sun.

As you start the diet, it would be good to remember that not everyone reacts to food in the same way. You should be careful to note how your body reacts to certain food. In addition, don't make any drastic changes, as this will prevent you from knowing which food is causing you problems. Also, remember that some foods may contain anti-inflammatory properties but they may also be high in unhealthy fat. It would be best to consume such foods in moderation.

Anti-Inflammatory Diet: What Not To Eat

When you're trying to reduce inflammation, you will achieve greater by knowing which foods to stay away from. Some foods are pro-inflammatory and frankly, most of them are just not good for your general health. Some of these foods include:

Sugar

Taking sugar increases your blood sugar levels and as we have learned, high insulin levels can trigger inflammation. In addition, sugar encourages your body to release cytokines. These are inflammatory messengers that lead to inflammation. Avoid sugar, soda and other sweet drinks.

Red meat

When you eat red meat, a chemical called NEu5gc is produced. When this happens, your body goes into an inflammatory immune response to deal with the chemical. Therefore, you would do well to avoid this. You should also try to avoid processed red meat such as hot dogs. These are usually high in saturated fat, which often causes inflammation especially when you eat too much red meat.

Dairy

Many people add milk to their breakfast cereal each morning. We also love having some cookies with a glass of milk. However, if you want to treat inflammation, you need to reduce your intake of milk. Why, you may ask. This is because milk has allergens such as casein, which spark inflammation.

Additionally, about 60% of the world's population are unable to digest milk in the first place. How many times do parents accuse their kids of eating 'too much' ice cream when they complain of having stomach cramps and feeling gassy. Guess what? It could just be that the kids are lactose intolerant.

Taking dairy products can lead to inflammatory responses such as hives, breathing difficulties, stomach distress, diarrhoea, constipation, acne, and skin rashes. These are clearly symptoms you can do away with by staying away from dairy products.

Trans-fats and excessive Omega 6 fatty acids

The ratio of omega 3 to omega 6 in your diet should be 1:1 or there about. Unfortunately, many people do not consume enough omega 3 fatty acids in their diet but take too much omega 6s for instance by using polyunsaturated fats such as sunflower, corn oil, soybean oil and safflower. It is said that many people consume omega 3s and omega 6s in the ration 1:20. This brings about an imbalance that leads to, cellular damage, inflammation and pain.

Similarly, many people consume trans fat. Hydrogenated and partially hydrogenated fats should have no business in your diet as they contribute largely to inflammation.

Refined Carbohydrates

Refined carbohydrates are grouped among the 'high glycemic index foods'. These are foods that lead to rapid increases in blood sugar (hyperglycemia). Hyperglycemia is often linked with inflammatory diseases. It triggers the release of cytokines which are inflammatory molecules.

On the other hand, when you eat carbohydrates that have natural fiber and fat, you will experience fewer pro-inflammatory agents. Stick to such carbohydrates instead of consuming refined carbohydrates.

Foods that cause allergies

Just because a certain food is known to work well in treating inflammation does not mean that it will work well for you. Some foods cause allergic reactions and initiate an inflammatory response. For example, some people are intolerant to dairy and wheat (gluten). Such people would do well to stay away from such foods. This is why it is wise to add one or two things to your diet at a time. This way, you can gauge your body's reaction to the foods you are including in your diet.

Knowing what to eat and what not to eat is just part of the journey towards reducing inflammation. The next step is actually using that knowledge to make the needed changes and achieve success.

Strategies To Put You On The Path To Success

It is one thing to know that you should add more fruits and vegetables in your daily diet but it is another thing to actually do it. This is especially so if you are used to eating high-carb foods and getting take-out. Fortunately, there are strategies you can use to improve your diet.

Figure out ways to sneak in anti-inflammatory foods

One way to increase your intake of anti-inflammatory foods is to incorporate them into your existing meals. This way, you will make your meals healthier without feeling as if you are making many changes at the same time. You can:

- Add foods such as celery, turmeric, and beetroot to your juice.

- Add garlic and turmeric to sauces.

- Add gibgerm flax oil, chia seeds and turmeric to your smoothies. You can also add avocado.

- Add quinoa to soups for added fiber and asparagus, beetroot, celery, cauliflower, ginger and turmeric to make soups more anti-inflammatory.

- If you're making a salad, take the opportunity to add various veggies and fruits. You can also add anti-inflammatory herbs such as ginger. Use oils such as flax oil for your dressing.

Make a transition plan

Quitting 'cold turkey' is quite difficult. In fact, many who do so soon find themselves back to their old habits because they cannot handle the changes. Instead of trying to get rid of everything at once, you can work out a transition plan that will get you to where you want to be. To do so:

- List down all the foods you eat and that you should give up. Once you list down such foods, determine which two foods you will give up each month. Then proceed to cut back on those two foods until you completely eliminate them from your diet. For example, if you want to reduce your intake of dairy, you can reduce your intake to 5 times a week, then three times, then once and finally you can remove dairy from your diet.

- List down all the foods you should eat and begin to add them to your diet. Remember you will be cutting down on foods you should not eat. When you do this, you can substitute the foods you shouldn't eat with those that you should eat. For example, after giving up refined carbs, you can start including whole grains in your diet. This way, your meals won't change but their quality will.

- Start drinking more water and eating healthier snacks. Also, you should start watching your portions to ensure you not only eat the needed foods but that you also eat enough of them to make a substantial change.

The idea is to make lifelong changes that will allow you to leave a healthy life without pain. You can do this by making small and deliberate changes and pretty soon you will have developed good eating habits to last a lifetime.

Look for new recipes

Adopting an anti-inflammatory diet will mean that you will have to start eating foods you are not used to. Since you will be eating new foods, you are likely to eat the same old foods over and over again. Eating the same foods day in day out can be boring; hence, the need to find new recipes that you can try out. This will expand your horizons and keep things interesting at the same time. You can dedicate at least one day per week to trying something you have not tried before. If you like it, add it to your diet.

Develop good eating habits

Eating habits are formed over time and they become so ingrained that you rarely think about them in detail. For example, you may find yourself always having coffee with toast for breakfast. It becomes your usual routine. Well, if you wish to be successful at reducing inflammation, you have to develop good eating habits that will allow you to do just that. One thing you can do is follow the anti-inflammatory diet pyramid developed by Dr. Joe Feuerstein (Columbia University). The pyramid indicates the foods you should eat starting from the bottom to the top level.

- Bottom level – Vegetables and fruits should feature prominently in your daily diet. Eat 2-3 fruits and 6-8 servings of veggies and salads every day.

- Level II - Whole grains and healthy carbs such as yams, plantains, whole grain pasta and quinoa should be eaten in limited amounts.

- Level III - Nuts and seeds should feature in your diet as should avocado, hemp and olive oils.

- Level IV - Proteins such as tofu, whole soy, tempeh, sardines, salmon, herring and sockeye should be eaten in moderation.

- Level V - This level includes foods such as eggs, bison, natural cheese and skinless poultry. These foods should be eaten in small amounts. Also, remember to remove the skin from any poultry you eat.

- Top level - The top level of the pyramid includes foods that you should eat in small amounts. These include things like dark chocolate and red wine.

When you change your eating habits to include various anti-inflammatory foods, you will start seeing the difference as you become healthier and pain-free. Forming a habit is a process. But it can be done and many have done it successfully, so can you. In addition, you can do other things to reduce inflammation.

Lower your calorie intake

Another thing that can help you address inflammation is reducing the amount of calories you eat. Eating fewer calories ensures you do away with diseases and conditions such as obesity, heart disease, type II diabetes. All these diseases have been linked to causing inflammation. A great way to reduce your calorie intake is to increase your vegetable intake and lower your intake of carbohydrates especially refined carbohydrates. This is because vegetables are high in fiber but very low in calories, which ensures you feel full. Vegetables are also rich in antioxidants. Therefore, when you increase your vegetable and fruit intake, you are taking foods rich in antioxidants, which will help in fighting inflammation.

Start Exercising

It is true that when you engage in bouts of exercise, your body experiences increased inflammation; you will suddenly find your joints and muscles aching. However, it is also true, if you continue engaging in regular exercise, you will be in the 'best shape' you've ever been in. This is because regular exercise decreases inflammation. Thus, instead of aiming high, you first need to lower your standards so that your body can get accustomed to the pace at which you are putting it through. As they say, don't run before you learn how to walk. Start by taking walks, increasing the distance and reducing the time for the walks. This way, your body will gradually adjust and before you know it, you will become fit and you will experience all the benefits that come with exercising.

Have adequate sleep

When you don't have enough sleep, you soon find yourself complaining of various ailments. The same goes when you sleep 'too much', you wake up with aching joints and complain of backaches among other ailments. When your sleep is disturbed, you also experience a variety of symptoms that bother you throughout the day. This clearly shows that the amount and quality of your sleep is linked to inflammation. Actually, insomnia and sleep disturbances increase the risk factor of inflammation.

Make sure that you get at least 7-8hours of uninterrupted sleep. Try coming up with a sleep schedule that will allow you to get the needed sleep. Set a night time routine and stick to it as much as you can so that your brain can adjust to the routine and prepare for sleep.

Keep a food journal

As we have said before, not all foods on the anti-inflammatory diet will be suitable for you. Additionally, other foods not on the list can actually be good for you. This means that you may have to take some time to figure out which foods are good for you. This is where a food journal comes in. You can write down what you're eating and how it makes you feel. This will enable you to find the foods that trigger inflammation. Thus, you will know the foods you should avoid and those that you can eat.

De-stress

Stress can only help you if it is a little and it drives you to action. However, when your body is in a constant state of stress, this just adds to inflammation and other undesired consequences. This is why it is important to de-stress.

The first thing you need to do is acknowledge that stress comes from various sources, and while you may not be able get rid of the sources of stress, there is still a lot you can do to minimize and manage the stress. As a rule, if you can change the situation, change it. If you cannot, accept it and find ways to deal with it. For example, if you have to deal with traffic each day on your way to work, you can listen to an audio book instead of focusing on the stressful situation. This will shift the focus to a more positive outcome.

Basically, your goal should be to try to find something you enjoy doing and set some few minutes aside to just doing it. That time alone will put you in a better mind frame.

Meditate

Meditation is one way you can reduce stress and help reduce inflammation. You do not need a complex routine in order to meditate. You can do simple breathing exercises where you focus on your breath as the air goes in through your nose and out through your mouth. Focus on the rise and fall of your stomach as you breathe. This will help you relax your mind and prepare you to deal with day-to-day situations.

To start meditating, set aside a few minutes and choose a quiet place where you can effectively meditate without distractions. If you find yourself distracted while you are meditating, don't beat yourself up. Just return your focus to your breathing.

Enjoy your social life

Your diet shouldn't dictate your social life. If it does, you may end up feeling resentful and breaking the rules. The truth is that everybody has to eat. This does not mean that you all have to eat at the same time. Thus, you can grab a bite before going to see your friends. This way, you can just have a salad that does not mess up with your diet.

Alternatively, you can make it a point to know which foods you can safely eat when you are out. This will make your work easier as you will have various options. You can also let your friends know that you are on the anti-inflammatory diet. This will stroke their curiosity and they will be more than happy to lookout for you and ensure you have no trouble finding something you can safely eat.

Establish a support system

A support system is like a comfort blanket. It shields you from negativity, props you up when you feel like giving up and listens to you when you want to lament about your problems. This is why many people starting a new diet, first try to establish a support system.

You can get a friend to try out the diet with you or have someone who will hold you accountable. This person can check to see if you have achieved certain goals. You can decide on a penalty and a reward system if you miss or achieve your goal. You can also have post-it notes with reminders of what you're doing and why it is important. This will keep you focused on your goal. Another thing you can do is join online forums. When you interact with like-minded people, you will get to share your journey and learn from their stories.

At the end of it all, what you are trying to do is change your lifestyle so that you can live a healthy life without pain. When you eat anti-inflammatory foods, drink a lot of water, exercise and sleep well, you are giving your body the best chance to fight inflammation. This in turn leads to a healthy pain free life.

In the following chapter, I will give you some sample anti-inflammatory recipes that you can try out.

Sample Recipes For Anti Inflammatory Diet

Breakfast
Gingerbread Oatmeal

Servings: 4

Ingredients

¼ teaspoon ground coriander

Maple syrup to taste

¼ teaspoon ground ginger

¼ teaspoon ground cardamom

¼ teaspoon ground allspice

1 cup steel cut oats

4 cups water

1 ½ tablespoons ground cinnamon

1 teaspoon ground cloves

1/8 teaspoon ground nutmeg

Instructions

Cook the oats according to instructions on the packet but add the spices when adding the oats into the water.

Once done, add some maple syrup to taste.

Serve and enjoy!

Apple and Ginger Muffins

Servings: 8

Ingredients

1 free-range egg

2 tablespoons finely chopped crystallised ginger

2 tablespoons organic corn flour

½ teaspoon ground cinnamon

¼ cup unrefined raw sugar

¼ cup olive oil

¼ cup brown rice flour

2 teaspoons gluten-free baking powder

1/3 cup + 1 tablespoon almond milk

½ cup almond meal (ground almonds)

1 teaspoon vanilla extract

1 cup finely sliced rhubarb

½ cup buckwheat flour

A pinch of sea salt

½ teaspoon ground ginger

1 apple, peeled, cored and finely diced

1 tablespoon ground linseed meal

Instructions

Preheat your oven to 350 degrees F.

Line 8 1/3 cup capacity muffin tins with paper cases or grease with oil.

Place the sugar, linseed meal, almond meal and ginger in a medium bowl and sieve in the spices, flours and baking powder and stir to combine thoroughly. Add in the apple and rhubarb and mix.

In a smaller bowl, whisk together the milk, egg, oil and vanilla then pour it directly into the flour mixture. Stir until just combined.

Divide the batter evenly between the paper cases or tins and scatter a few slices of rhubarb if desired.

Bake in the oven for about 20 to 25 minutes or until golden around the edges and risen.

Remove from the oven and let it cool for 5 minutes before transferring to a wire rack to cool completely.

Eat while warm or at room temperature.

You can store in an airtight container for 3 to 5 days or for longer frozen in Ziploc bags.

Lunch Recipes
Mediterranean Tuna Salad

Servings: 2

Ingredients

2 large vine-ripened tomatoes

2, 5 ounce cans tuna packed in water, drained

Salt and pepper

¼ cup chopped kalamata or mixed olives

2 tablespoons chopped fire roasted red peppers

1 tablespoon capers

¼ cup mayonnaise

1 tablespoon fresh lemon juice

2 tablespoons chopped fresh basil

2 tablespoons minced red onion

Instructions

Add all the ingredients except the tomatoes into a large bowl and stir to combine.

Chop the tomatoes into sixths but don't cut them all the way through and gently pull open.

Scoop the tuna salad into the centre.

Serve and enjoy!

Note

You can also serve the salad as a sandwich, on a bed of greens or with some crackers.

Scale back the sodium by reducing the amount of olives and capers.

Winter Fruit Salad

Servings: 6

Ingredients

¾ cup pecans- cut into half lengthwise

4 Fuyu persimmons cut into 1 inch cubes

1 cup grapes, cut into halves

3 Bosch pears, chopped into 1 inch cubes

Dressing Ingredients:

1 tablespoon peanut oil

1 tablespoon extra virgin olive oil

1 tablespoon pomegranate- flavoured vinegar

2 tablespoons agave nectar

Pinch of salt- to taste

Instructions

Whisk together all the dressing ingredients in a bowl and let it sit as you prepare the fruits

Toss the fruits with the dressing and just before you serve toss with the pecan pieces.

Enjoy!

Note

You could use other fruits such as figs or apples; just make sure you have about 5 to 6 cups of cut fruit in total.

Dinner Recipes
Slow Cooker Turkey Chilli

Servings 8-10

Ingredients

1 red pepper, chopped

1 tablespoon cumin

1 medium onion, diced

1 pound 99% lean ground turkey

1 tablespoon olive oil

1 cup frozen corn

1 (16 ounces) jar sliced jalapeno peppers, drained

Salt and black pepper- to taste

2 (15 ounces) cans red kidney beans, rinsed and drained

2 (15 ounces) cans petite diced tomatoes

2 (15 ounces) cans black beans, rinsed and drained

1 yellow pepper, chopped

2 (15 ounces) cans tomato sauce

2 tablespoons chili powder

Optional toppings: green onions, shredded cheese, avocado, sour cream/ Greek yogurt

Instructions

Add oil to a skillet over medium heat.

Add the turkey to the skillet and cook until brown then transfer turkey to slow cooker.

Add the peppers, diced tomatoes, jalapenos, chilli powder, onion, tomato sauce, beans, corn and cumin into the cooker and season with pepper and salt and stir.

Cover and cook on high for about 4 hours or for 6 hours on low.

Serve with the toppings- if desired.

Note

Reduce the sodium content by going for fresh jalapenos and choosing low sodium canned beans.

Kale Salad with Grilled Chicken Wrap

Servings: 2

Ingredients

6 cups curly kale, cut into bite sized pieces

1/8 cup olive oil

¾ cup finely shredded Parmesan cheese

½ coddled egg (cooked about 1 minute)

1 clove garlic, minced

½ teaspoon Dijon mustard

1 cup cherry tomatoes, quartered

1/8 cup fresh lemon juice

1 teaspoon honey or agave

2 Lavash flat breads or two large tortillas

Kosher salt and freshly ground black pepper

8 ounces grilled chicken, thinly sliced

Instructions

Mix half the coddled egg, mustard, lemon juice, minced garlic, honey and olive oil in a bowl and whisk to make the dressing. Season with some salt and pepper to taste.

Add the chicken, cherry tomatoes and chicken and toss to coat with the dressing and a quarter cup of the shredded parmesan.

Spread out 2 lavash flatbreads and evenly distribute the salad over the warps and sprinkle ¼ cup parmesan to each.

Roll up the wraps, slice in half and enjoy!

I need your help..

We have come to the end of the book. Thank you for reading and congratulations for reading until the end.

As you have learned, an anti-inflammatory diet is meant to stop or reduce inflammation. It does this by including foods rich in antioxidants and fiber and other anti-inflammatory properties. Fruits, vegetables, whole grains, fish and seafood are some of the foods you can use to reduce inflammation. In addition, reducing inflammation will help you reduce pain associated with inflammation and you can live a healthy life free of pain.

Finally, if you enjoyed this book, would you be kind enough to leave a review for this book on Amazon? It'd be greatly appreciated!

I want to reach as many people as I can with this book, and more reviews will help me accomplish that!

Thank you and good luck!

Preview Of '20 Easy And Fast Diet Tips For Losing Weight'

Before we start learning about the strategies you can use to lose weight, let's start by highlighting some of the benefits that will come as a result of shedding those extra pounds just to give you extra motivation to want to do something NOW.

Why You Need To Lose Weight

Healthy weight loss has over one hundred benefits; these include emotional and physical benefits. I will dedicate this section to discussing the health benefits that many people (and weight loss/health books) do not pay enough attention to.

1: You Avoid Pre-Diabetes or Type 2 Diabetes

Pre-diabetes/high blood glucose is a condition that develops when the blood sugar levels in your blood move past normal ranges but not enough to qualify as diabetes. When your body stops consistently producing insulin sufficient to meet your body's needs, or the amount produced does not work properly, type 2 diabetes is likely to develop. Being pre-diabetic places you at a very high risk of developing type 2 diabetes.

Being obese or overweight is a proven leading risk factor for type 2 diabetes because carrying excess weight typically makes it hard for cells to respond to insulin, and since the additional fat acts as an insulating layer, it makes it more difficult for the sugar to enter the cells, which results in more circulating blood sugar levels.

Nonetheless, if you are already a pre-diabetic, you can prevent the progression to diabetes by shedding some weight (to reduce the insulating layer on cells so that they respond more to insulin) and trying to maintain a healthy weight.

2: You Keep Your Heart Healthy

When it comes to heart disease, some of the key risk factors are high cholesterol and high blood pressure. Research shows that:

1. Excessive accumulation of body fat makes your body release particular chemicals that occur naturally into the bloodstream, which increases blood pressure, and

2. Being overweight makes the liver produce too much amounts of Low density Lipoprotein (LDL) also called cholesterol. LDL tends to be sticky and gathers in the walls of blood vessels, which causes the narrowing of arteries, a condition called atherosclerosis, which increases your risk of strokes and heart attack.

When you lose weight, your blood pressure often reduces and the liver naturally reduces the amount of LDL it produces.

Royal Adelaide Hospital conducted a research on cardiovascular improvements with respect to a special weight loss program. Their results showed a decrease of cholesterol by 12%, a 10% decrease of LDL, a 5% decrease in diastolic blood pressure, and an 8% decrease in systolic blood pressure.

3: Improved Sleep (and Possible Treatment of Sleep Apnea)

One of the most prominent benefits of losing weight is improved sleep. When you gain excess weight, you gather more soft tissues in the neck; this intensifies the incidence of snoring.

NOTE: Snoring is a result of constricted airways, which obstructs air movement.

Snoring can be a symptom of sleep apnea, a possible life-threatening condition characterized by obstruction of breathing that requires the victim to wake up frequently from sleep to resume breathing.

As a victim of sleep apnea, you rarely remember anything about the episodes of waking many times a night to breathe but even so, this sleep and oxygen deprivation could easily lead to a weak immune system, high blood pressure, heart disease, memory problems, and sexual dysfunction.

When you lose weight, you reduce the amount of fatty tissue in the back of your throat, decrease snoring and the likelihood of the worsening of your health- as aforementioned. You encourage better sleep quality and reduce the risk of developing sleep apnea.

4: Better Joints (Mobile and Pain-Free)

Osteoarthritis (OA) is one of the most common joint disorders. It causes the tissues that protect the joints (cartilage and bone) to wear away. Consequently, the joints become tender and swollen, thus making movement very painful.

When you are overweight, you add to the load placed on the joints that bear the weight such as hips and knees.

NOTE: When you walk, you exert a force of approximately 3-6 times your entire body weight across the knee (read more on this page (check the discussion section) or here), so adding about 10 kg of weight does increase the force on the knees, which is equal to carrying 30-60 kgs^2 extra.

Therefore, a loss of merely 5% of your body weight could reduce the amount of stress placed on the knees, lower back, and hips, and reduce the pain (remember that losing 5kgs is equal to relieving a force of 15-30kgs^2 on the knees). According to doctors, a 10% loss of bodyweight has presented a 28% improvement in knee osteoarthritis symptoms.

Check out the rest of 20 Easy And Fast Diet Tips For Losing Weight on Amazon, go to: http://amzn.to/2mNtPEg

Check Out My Other Books

Below you'll find some of my other popular books that are popular on Amazon and Kindle as well.

Alternatively, you can visit my author page on Amazon to see other work done by me.

Ketogenic Cookbook: Quick Low Calorie Ketogenic Crockpot Recipes with 7 Days Meal Plan

Freedom: How to Make Money Online and Become Financially Free by Creating Passive Income

Mediterranean Diet: Instant Pot Cookbook with Delicious Recipes

Alice the Superbug

Madison and Astrid's first magical journey

Intermittent Fasting: The Essential Beginners Guide for Women for Weight Loss

Chakra Healing: Chakra Healing and Karmic Awareness for Beginners

SEO 2017 for Growth: The Ultimate Guide to Learn Search Engine Optimization with Internet Marketing Tips

Psychology: How to Analyze People Using Human Psychological Techniques, Body Language Signals, Social Skills and Personality Types

Paleo Smoothies: Recipes to Energize and for Ultimate Health and Weight Loss

Belly Diet Smoothies: Delicious Smoothie Recipes to Flatten Your Belly, Improve Your Gut & Burn Fat

Keto Diet: Keto Diet Guide Cookbook for Beginners with Meal Plan and Simple, Delicious Recipes to Lose Weight and Look Good

Online Business from Scratch: The 9 Step Guide to Building a Profitable and Sustainable Online Business

Weight Loss: 20 Easy And Fast Diet Tips For Losing Weight - An Easy-To-Follow Weight Loss Guide

Ketogenic Cookbook: Ketogenic Cookbook for Beginners with 7 Days Meal Plan

Negative Calorie Diet: Cookbook & Guide Which Will Help You To Burn Body Fat, Lose Weight And Live Healthy

Negative Calorie Diet with Anti-Inflammatory Diet Guide

Make Money Online To Achieve Freedom

Negative Calorie Diet with Smart Fat Guide

Negative Calorie Diet & Clean Eating: Cookbook & Guide Which Will Help You To Burn Body Fat, Lose Weight And Live Healthy

Smart Fat: Cookbook with Fat Meals Which Help You to Lose Weight, Get Healthy and Improve Brain Function

Anti-Inflammatory Diet Guide: The Guide to Reduce Inflammation and Live a Healthy Life Without Pain

Essential Oils: The Young Living Book Guide of Natural Remedies for Beginners for Pets, For Dogs

Clean Eating: Cookbook and Guide to Restore Your Body's Natural Balance and Eat Healthy

Anti-Inflammatory Diet Guide: The Guide to Reduce Inflammation and Live a Healthy Life Without Pain

Dash Diet: Cookbook for Weight Loss with Action Plan and Easy Recipes

Air Fryer Cookbook: Quick, Healthy and Easy Low Carb Air Fryer Recipes

Psychology & Habits Of Highly Effective People Box Set

Leptin Resistance: Leptin Diet to Control Your Hormones, Get Permanent Weight Loss, Cure Obesity and Live Healthy

Negative Calorie Diet & Dash Diet Box Set

Negative Calorie Diet & Weight Loss Box Set

Habits of Highly Effective People: What Are the Habits of Successful People?

Slow Cooker: Cookbook with Slow Cooker Recipes

Weight Loss Cookbook: Meal Prep Cookbook for Weight Loss and Clean Eating

Weight Loss Cookbook: Mediterranean Diet for Lasting Weight Loss

Negative Calorie Diet & Dash Diet Box Set

Slow Cooker & Instant Pot Box Set

Children Books: Madison and Astrid's first magical journey & Alice the Superbug Box Set

Belly Diet: The Zero Belly Diet Step-By-Step Guide Which Helps You to Lose Your Belly and Enjoy Your Flat Belly

Weight Loss: 20 Easy and Fast Diet Tips for Losing Weight - An Easy-To-Follow Weight Loss Guide

Instant Pot: Instant Pot Pressure Cooker Cookbook with Easy and Healthy Recipes

Vegan Cookbook: Vegan Cookbook For Beginners, For Kids And For Teens For Diabetics With Pictures

Low Carb: Low Carb Diet Cookbook with Low Carb Keto Recipes for Batch Cooking

Ketogenic Cooking: Ketogenic Cooking With Your Instant Pot

Passive Income: Passive Income Tutorial with 7 Online Ideas to Generate Passive Income Streams for Beginners

Low Carb Diet: Low Carb Diet Recipes Cookbook for Beginners for Batch Cooking

Bonus: Subscribe To The Free Weight Loss Report

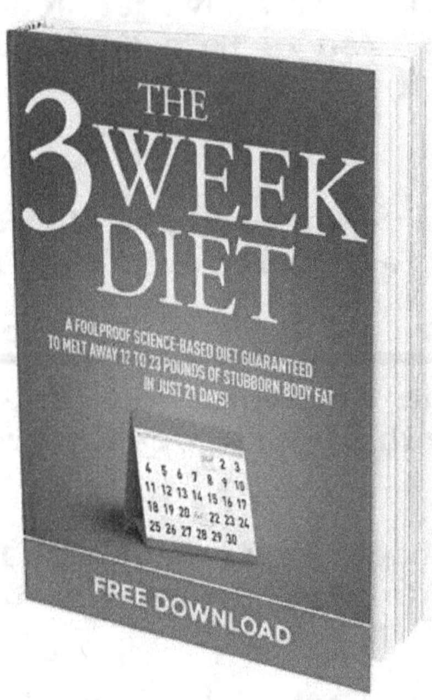

The Introduction Manual is more than just an introduction to the diet. Instead, it discusses the science behind how we gain and lose weight as well as what absolutely needs to be done to attack that stubborn body fat that, until now, has been so challenging to get rid of.

Here are the preview of what you'll get:

- Rapid Weight Loss
- How This System Works
- Why This Diet
- Why 3 Weeks?
- 21 Days To Make A Habit
- Fat Loss VS. Weight Loss
- Nutrients
- Protein, Fat, Carbohydrates
- The Food Pyramid And Obesity
- Fiber
- Metabolism
- How We Get Fat
- Triglycerides
- How To Get Thin
- Diet Overview
- Meal Frequency
- Water
- Diet Essentials
- Let's Get Started

To get instant access to these incredible ebook, go to:

http://bit.ly/2tUb9cp

9 781722 027605